Homemade Antibiotics:

Most Effective Remedies to Prevent and Cure Your Body With 100% Natural Components

Table of Content:

Introduction

Since I was a kid my immune system is really low that is why I always get various infectious diseases from time to time and it is really annoying already because I was too tired of going back and forth to the hospital. As I grew up I was still experiencing those kinds of dilemmas that is why I was really immune already with the usual antibiotics and I felt that I am only getting sicker that is why I came up with a decision that would change my life forever.

I came across learning how to make my own antibiotics and the most exciting is all of it is natural. It really fascinated me to know the different antibiotic ingredients that will help me manage my infectious diseases and most of all to make my life better.

Since then I was able to combat my different sicknesses effectively and the greatest thing is I did not experience any side-effects from it. Right now, I am completely healed after consuming the natural antibiotics that I have created. I can say that I am better than ever because I am really energized and feel like 10 years younger.

People were surprised when they saw the new me because they only know the former me which is weakling. I was really thankful that I found the natural antibiotics that I will introduce to you later. Since then I am never worried anymore if I get sick because I was always ready and I do not have to buy any more in the drug store because the ingredients are already present in my kitchen.

So I am proud to impart my knowledge to you regarding how to make your own natural antibiotics at the comforts of your own home. You will surely be amazed how powerful our nature is because the treatment that you needed are just there sitting on your kitchen and the effectiveness of it will not be compromised just like what you expect on the traditional antibiotics.

I suggest that you read this book meticulously so that you will make the most out of each ingredient. Your time will surely worth it while you are reading this wonderful book that is written with lots of love.

Chapter 1 – The Essence of Natural Antibiotics

It is given that every once in a while we are experiencing illnesses and most of the time it is all about infection. This is the primary reason why our doctors are prescribing us various types of antibiotics however it is really not advisable especially if the condition is not that worst simply because it can impose a significant amount of risk on your health due to side-effects that is why it is always better if you will have some alternative.

Thankfully, there are natural antibiotics available that you can create by yourself and you will be surprised how easy it is to make despite that it sounds super intimidating. However, expect that you should learn it first tremendously but do not worry because we will tackle a lot of natural antibiotics in this book.

But before we start tackling the ingredients and other stuff I would like to give you an insight into the benefits that you can get from natural antibiotics. Here are the benefits below.

- You will not experience any digestion problems and nausea because of natural antibiotics are very gentle and not harsh on our stomach.

- It will make not affect your appetite especially if you take the antibiotics between meals.

- It is much cheaper compared to the traditional medical antibiotics that are why you will surely save some money from it.

- You can battle out various infections in your body and at the same time promote better overall health because of the natural ingredients that the antibiotics are composed of.

- You will help your body to become immune in certain infectious diseases that could be fatal if taken for granted.

Aside from that there are other more benefits that you can get from it and if we will list them down all, this book is surely not enough to accommodate it and that is how amazing natural antibiotics are really great.

A Brief Background

Natural treatments utilized for several years already have several medicinal plants for recovering from a lot of ailments. Our forefathers usually mixed medicinal plants with some top-secret recipes that have been passed down to them generations by generations.

On the traditional way of healing, the skill were verbally passed regarding systems about cultivating plants, systems of getting ready, practice, dosage, routines and etc.

Since our facts about the importance of natural products in curing infectious diseases has not elevated so rapidly as researches on the sprout of modern antibiotics, but the appearance of multi-drug resistant types need the latest therapeutic methodologies.

Knowing the improvement of antibiotic resistance denoted difficult because there are lots of reasons involved such as genetic adaptation. Right now, we usually discover ourselves in a jeopardy selecting efficient treatment for infections.

Rest assured that bacteria have tremendously adapted their security to their outside forces and any latest genuine antibacterial substances will be outdated in the future.

Since the early ages, humans are battling with ailments particularly infections such as mild UTIs to serious illnesses. It is given that they used their instincts which allow them to use herbs that are present in their surroundings to cure their ailments.

The specific history of healing with plants on where it came from has diminished on the start of modern human's era. Humans have always attempted to get a grasp and treat the ailments, just as they have attempted to get a grasp of the man and nature correlation with each other.

We might tell that they deal with diseases in an instinctive manner, knowing the reasons and cures in everything with regards to wellbeing. In ancient times, humans were alert, persevered and the instance was considered differently. They were keen observers of the surroundings and were capable to create a great link among the tiniest details.

How early people, even they did not have any medical apparatus or supplies, crafted different methods that were unexplainable of modern science. An initial look of the early lifestyle of humans is that they are completely mobile as a matter of fact several remarkable feats are just like they were able to utilize the local products to produce their natural treatments.

There is a contest that plants and animal outputs were commonly utilized with more or less preciseness. For the majority of them, significant researches showed their medical functionalities. Many doctors included a unique border among allopathic, complementary and alternative healing introducing the increase of reductionist way or, opposite, the all-natural ways.

For a short instance, there is an increase in equal point of views in determining the effective aspects of those methodologies and making the most out of them. Precise researches about the preciseness of natural medicine ways of healing are only little but still the upward thinking of people on this methodology, even for medical patients, will, surely able us to think about it more.

Also, studies on plant extracts with antibacterial processes have been known to search proof that tells plants importance in contagious diseases. To prove that natural antibiotics are already there since the early ages one example is the phytotherapy because if not the earliest technique, utilized in curing of infectious diseases it is absolutely the first one invented.

Many nations have a custom in a natural way of healing as individuals in nations where alternative medicine is popular are more acquainted to pursing these doings. These days, natural healers are attempting to cure infectious diseases such as HIV with the use of plant extracts minus the fact of their effectiveness.

Also, several strains of antibiotic plants are aggressive, to sum it up the lack of success of antibiotic treatment may be the outcome of a known gentle plant extract just like a rose.

All over the globe, there are lots of facts diminished about traditional medicine, regarding the use of plants and how people used it to their advantage. Phytotherapy utilizes the whole plant or portions of plants getting readied by different techniques.

Right now, there are lots of plant outputs—oils, colors, extracts, powders, and etc. There are researches that not only show the antibacterial output of several plants but also check the prospected target of the action.

The Downsides Of Natural Antibiotics

Even if a product has a sign that telling it is all-natural, it is not always harmless. The content of dynamic ingredients differs depends on its brand. Check the labels meticulously. An individual should also tell their doctor if they want to consume any natural antibiotics.

Even garlic is commonly harmless when eaten, studies depict that consuming pure garlic may heighten the occurrence of bleeding. This can be harmful to individuals that will undergo surgery. Pure garlic may also lessen the effect of HIV drugs.

You should keep away from certain substances such as colloidal silver because it has small pieces of silver if put in water.

Colloidal silver is suggested as a cure for different illnesses, such as STDs and bubonic plague. Consuming colloidal silver might obstruct with the efficiency of anti-inflammatory and drugs utilized to cure a nonperforming thyroid gland. Silver can accumulate inside our system and make our skin pale which is called argyria.

When Should You Utilize Antibiotic Drugs?

Antibiotics might be utilized to quicken rejuvenation from sickness or to stop the multiplication of contagious diseases. Because of the recent elevation in illnesses that are resistant to prescription medicines a lot of medical professionals do not suggest the use of antibiotics unless they are efficient and needed.

Antibiotics are usually used to treat:

- Stop the accumulation of contagious diseases – because they inhibit the growth of bacteria which will stop the spread of sicknesses.

- Stop the condition from worsening the condition – since you will stop the bacteria from spreading you will surely control the illness.

- Quicken up the healing from injury or sickness – it puts up some sort of protective coating on your immune system that will let the injury or sickness heal much quicker.

- Stop complications from happening – because you will already take action on the disease itself expect that complications will not rise up.

- If an individual is taking artificial antibiotics, they must consume the whole dosage as suggested. This is specifically made for individuals with an elevated risk of bacterial infection, or is expected to become ill because of some conditions that they already have namely:

- Will undergo surgery – it will help them minimize the chances of complications that might happen because of surgery.

- Undergoing chemotherapy treatment – since chemotherapy weakens the immune system, patients are suspected to accumulate viral infections much easier compared to normal individuals.

- HIV problems – it is known that HIV is an infection that is caused by a specific virus, high dosage of antibiotics is much recommended.

- Currently, on treatment for diabetes – diabetic patients are susceptible to infection if they have wounds that is why antibiotics are given to help them cope up with their wounds and etc.

- Heart-disease problems – it is advisable for them to take the complete dosage at all times because wrong amounts of dosage can make them immune to it and future illnesses can increase their risk of compromising their health.

- Recovering from wounds – antibiotics are very crucial for wounds because they promote healing and prevents the bacteria from spreading which promotes quicker recovery.

- Senior citizens – since they are already in their old age they are pretty delicate to the wrong dosage of antibiotics that is why it is strictly suggested that senior citizens must ensure that their antibiotic intake is correct at all times.

- Below 3 days of age – a very delicate individual when it comes to antibiotic consumption that is why ensure that the pediatrician is credible and you must follow the medical advice given meticulously.

When a person is suspected in allergens to artificial antibiotics they may be urged to talk their alternatives with a medical professional. Simply because there are people that are quite sensitive to any sorts of medications that is why you must also make sure that you are not in the category that is why you must always feel yourself for that sort of condition.

Chapter 2 – Homemade Antibiotics For Viral Infection

Several organic products have anti-inflammatory functionalities, but which are not hazardous to utilize, and when should an individual utilize them?

Artificial antibiotics just like penicillin, have supported humans to recuperate from critical illnesses for several decades already. But, humans are also substituting those artificial ways to natural ways for various reasons.

Research has shown that 2 out of 20 people are getting some side effects that are very annoying for the digestive system after consuming antibiotics. Some of them also experience some allergies because of it

In this subchapter, we check the proofs behind some of the greatest natural antibiotics. So let us not delay the learning and let us start!

Garlic

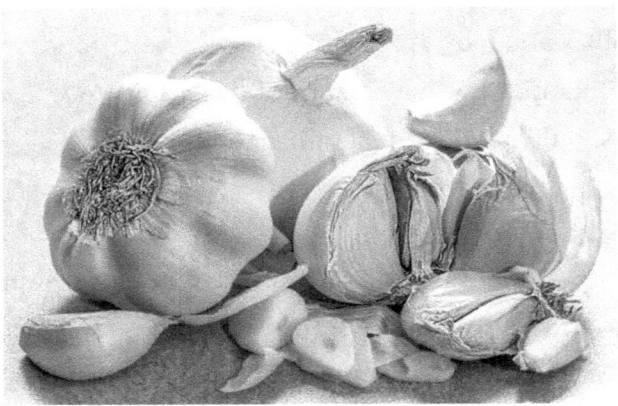

It is known as a proven treatment to combat bacteria. The medical doctors and scientists are still skeptical about the use of such natural technique as an antibiotic. While individuals have utilized useful objects like these for thousands of years already as a large number of treatments have not completely undergone a significant amount of tests.

But several pieces of them depict remarkable outcome with the continuous use of it. There is a current elevation in medicine-resistant organisms experts are searching to the natural way of intervention in creating new medicines.

Furthermore, various individuals and ethnic groups globally have known garlic for its wondrous effects. The study has discovered that garlic is a great solution to combat various forms of organisms that harm human health. It is also known to utilize on tuberculosis which is also a dreadful disease.

See? Garlic is not just your regular ingredient at your kitchen because it has lots of advantages when used in natural treatments.

Honey

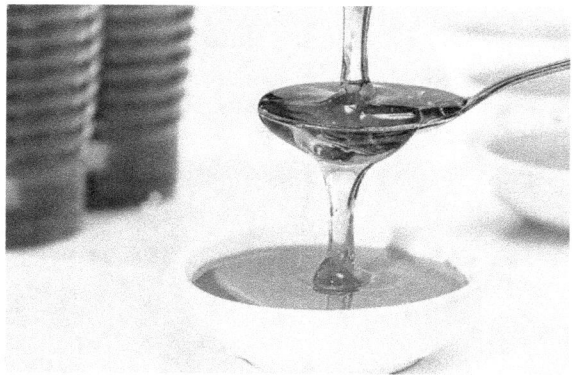

Since ancient times, honey has been utilized as an ointment that cures wounds and avoids inflammation to happen. Experts today have discovered it beneficial in curing burns, wounds, and other types of painful wounds. For instance, there is a successful study that shows honey to speed up wound healing.

The anti-inflammatory outcomes of honey are commonly related to its hydrogen peroxide substance. But, manuka honey battles bacteria, though it has a lesser hydrogen peroxide substance. It also gives a coating for security that promotes a humid setting.

Ginger

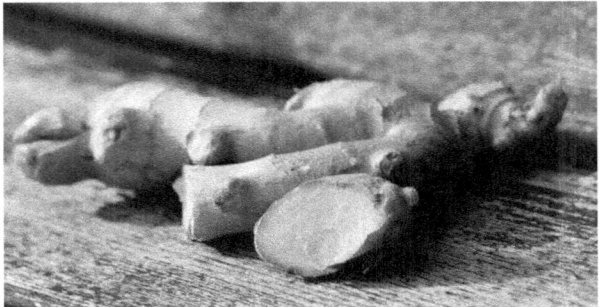

The experts also depict ginger as natural anti-bacterial medicine. Various researches have shown that ginger's capacity to battle out various types of bacteria.

Experts are also finding out the ginger's power to combat nausea and seasickness as well as to minimize blood sugar.

Goldenseal

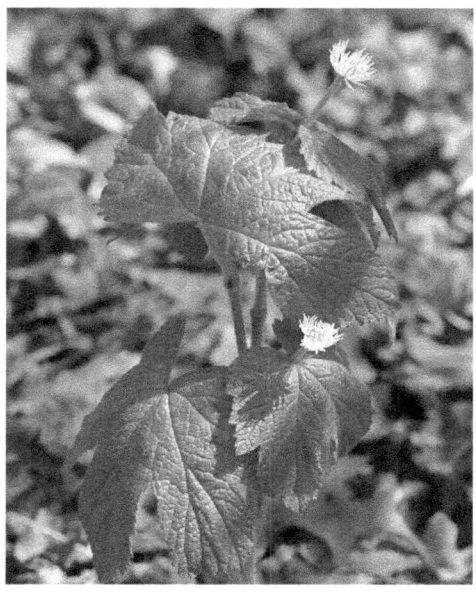

It is commonly taken as a capsule or tea to heal digestive and respiratory issues. But, it might also fight UTI and loose bowel movement. Moreover, outputs of new research help the utilization of goldenseal to cure skin problems. An individual that is consuming artificial drugs should go to a doctor before consuming goldenseal, as this goldenseal can result in the intrusion.

Goldenseal also has berberine, a crucial ingredient of natural antibiotics. This alkaloid is not supposed to be used for pregnant women and infants. It can be purchased easily because lots of health stores are selling them.

Elderberry

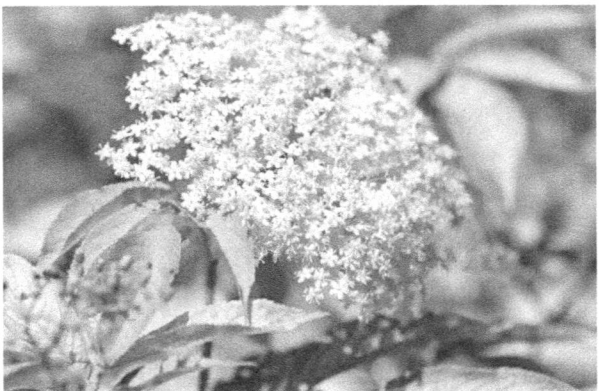

The usual black elderberry has been utilized to lessen the stages of flu symptoms. By consuming 50 milliliters per day for adults and 20 ml for kids support a healthy rejuvenation of your immune system, in just less than 2 days.

This content blends to the small spikes on a germ protein that are utilized to get through and occupy healthy cells and ruins them so that the virus is inefficient. It might also be great to battle out herpes and other types of viruses.

Echinacea

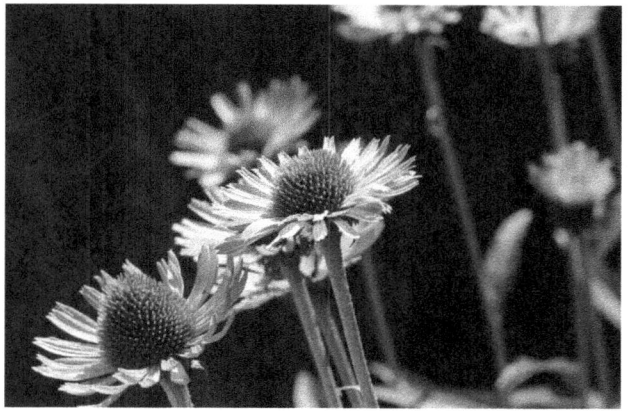

This natural antibiotic is amazing for the immune system and has a straightforward anti-bacterial solution to battle out bronchitis and colds. The leaves and tops are the ones that are utilized the latter are the most efficient at supporting the system to get rid of the viruses.

Green Tea

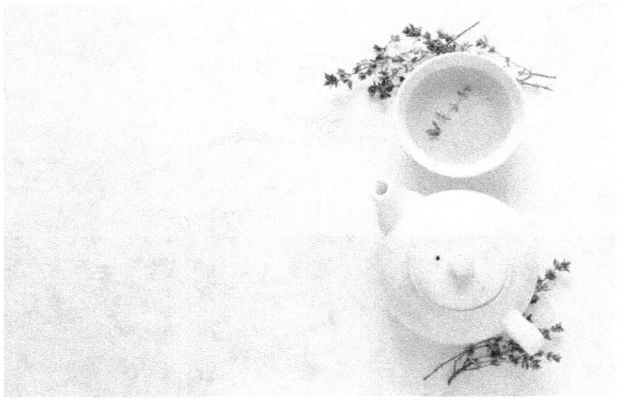

It contains flavonoids known as catechins, which is known to stopping viral infections by stopping the enzymes that give it the privilege to multiply. Green tea has been recognized to be efficient in inhibiting hepatitis B and certain STDs.

Licorice

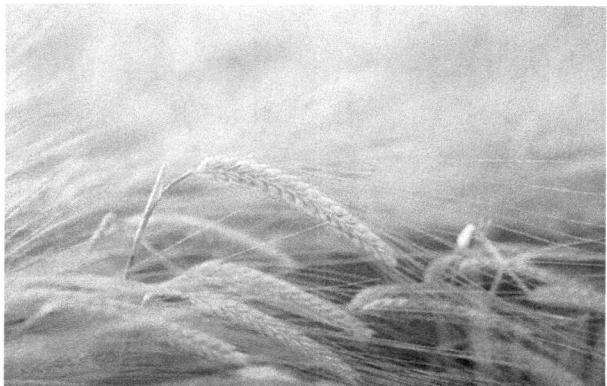

It has a content known as glycyrrhizin that lessens the multiplication of infection and stops the capacity to get inside and multiply on human's healthy cells. It is also recognized to be great in curing various viral diseases such as hepatitis and other viral infections.

Hypericum perforatum

It is also recognized for its capacity to heal certain viral infection as well as emotional problems. It also contains substances that combat viruses that work by mimicking already present cells through "camouflaging".

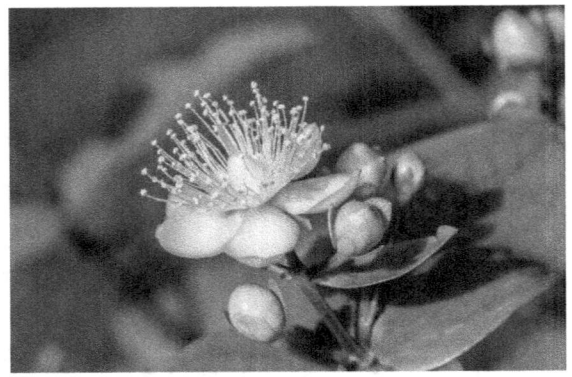

These viruses that cover-ups as human cells are hepatitis and STDs. For a more desirable outcome, it is suggested that you can use more than 1 dosage of those to diminish viruses.

Olive Leaf

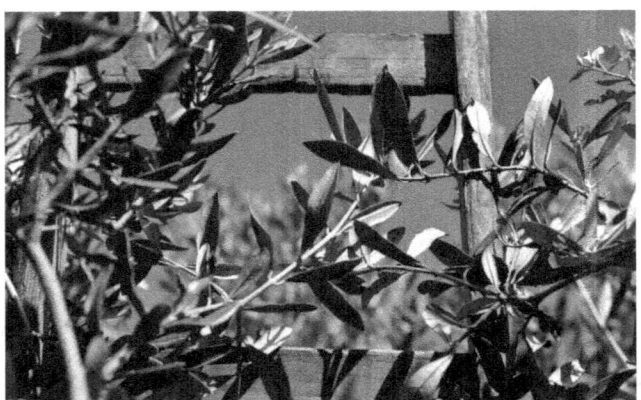

Its leaves have contents known as calcium elonate and elenoic acid that has been proven to be a great terminator of many viruses such as herpes, influenza, coxsackie, and polioviruses. These factors stop the multiplication of enzymes that gives viruses the ability to reproduce.

Pau D'Arco

It is also known as ipe roxo or lapacho, is an Amazon tree that possesses inner bark that can cure a lot of viral infections such as colds, flu, herpes, and STDs. It has quinoids that stop virus replication by destroying the DNA inside the virus that would blend itself in a well-sound human cell and multiply.

Clove

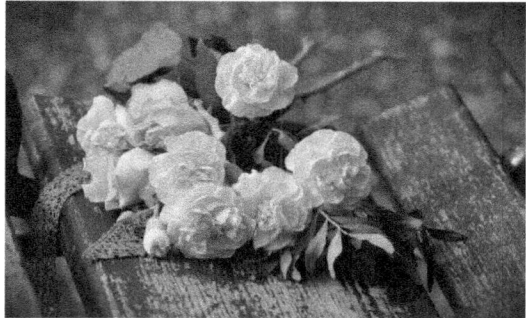

It is commonly have been utilized in the dental industry.
A study is now searching that clove water extract might be
good versus various types of bacteria just like E. coli.

Oregano

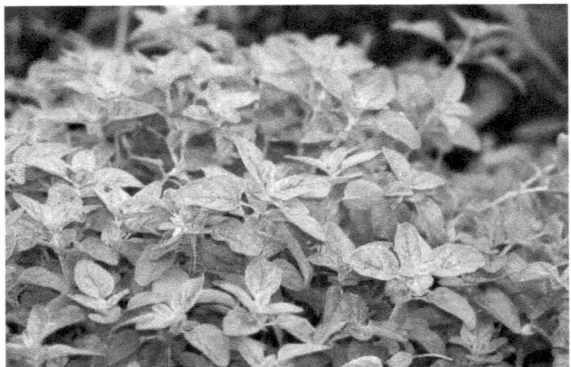

Some people have the notion that oregano helps the
immune system to become strong and performs as an
antioxidant. It may possess anti-inflammatory substances.

What I loved about these natural antibiotics is that they do
not only cure my viral infection but they also strengthen my
immune system as well. This why among all the other
categories of natural antibiotics these are my most favorite.

Chapter 3 – DIY Antibiotics for Stomach Issues

Stomach ulcers are exposed openings within the surface of the stomach. On the other hand, stomach flu has almost the same symptoms of diarrhea which are stomach pain, loose bowel movement, nausea and etc.

The usual root of stomach ulcers is the strain of bacteria which is called H.Pylori. Stomach flu and ulcers are healed with prescription antibiotics to lessen and stop stomach acid from flowing.

Furthermore to this effective treatment routine, studies have revealed that there are several natural treatments that might be beneficial in helping you cope up with stomach flu and ulcer.

Flavonoids

Those are compounds that sprout in nature in many veggies and fruits. Foods and drinks loaded in flavonoids are:

- ✓ berries

- ✓ soybeans
- ✓ apples
- ✓ red grapes
- ✓ legumes
- ✓ kale
- ✓ teas
- ✓ broccoli

These nourishments might support the body as well in battling versus the H. pylori strain. Those foods will help you protect the surface of the stomach and could make the ulcers to recover.

The advantageous thing is that there are no side effects of eating flavonoids that are present in the traditional diet, but heightened amounts of flavonoids might be responsible for blood clotting.

Deglycyrrhizinated licorice

Despite its long name, it is just the same simple old licorice with an extra sweetness. Research depicts that deglycyrrhizinated licorice supports the diminishing of ulcers by stopping the spread of H. pylori.

You cannot acquire this outcome from consuming licorice candy and excessive consumption of licorice candy can be harmful to certain individuals. Eating more than 2 oz. every day for half a month can turn heart issues or hypertension worse.

Probiotics

Probiotics are a combination of alive yeast and bacteria that will give you overall wellness and crucial microorganisms to your digestive system. Probiotics can be found on the traditional foods that we eat such as fermented foods.

- o yogurt
- o kimchi
- o buttermilk
- o miso
- o kefir

Research depicts that probiotics might get rid of H. pylori and elevate the healing rate for individuals with stomach flu and ulcers when supplemented to the conventional routine of antibiotics.

Honey

Reliant on its source, honey can comprise of hundreds of elements, which comprise of polyphenols and lots of antioxidants. It is also a powerful solution against bacterial infection and effective in preventing H. pylori growth.

Until blood sugar levels get high, you can utilize honey just like any other sweeteners that you use but the good thing is it is beneficial for your stomach.

Cranberry

It is known is some researches to support the diminishing UTIs by stopping bacteria from accumulating on the surfaces of the bladder. H.Pylori is also weak when it comes to contact with a cranberry. You have the ability to consume cranberry on different forms such as food, drinks, and supplements. No exact number of consumption is linked with a cure.

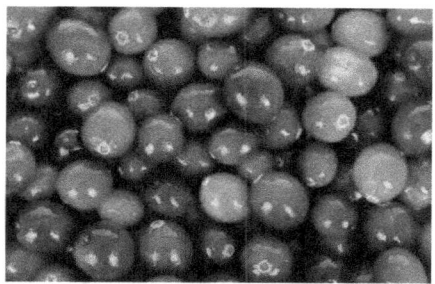

However, excess cranberry consumption in any type may result in stomach and intestinal issues because of its elevated sugar content, so initiate with little amounts and slowly heighten your consumption.

Many over-the-counter cranberry juices are extremely sweetened with sweeteners, which can also put up empty kcals. Keep out from those beverages by purchasing juice that is flavored naturally.

Mastic

It came from a tree's sap that is usually grown in the Mediterranean. Researches have shown the efficiency of this on H. pylori issues varied, but there is research that tells that consuming a gum made out of this might get rid of H. pylori which promotes better overall health particularly on our digestive tract.

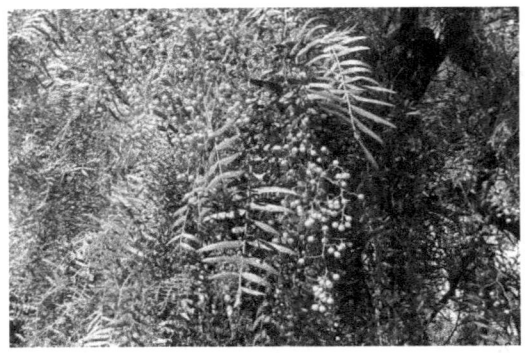

But, based on the conventional treatments that medical professionals advice the gum was greatly less efficient than drugs. The conventional cure diminished the bacteria in more than half of the samples studied.

Fruits, veggies, and whole grains

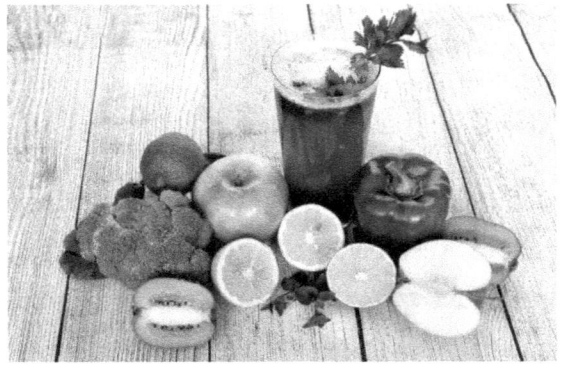

A diet focused on fruits, veggies, and whole grains is not only excellent for your overall wellbeing. The reason for this is that a nutritious diet can support your system to cure your ulcer.

Foods possessing the polyphenols may help you prevent or heal ulcers and other stomach-related problems. You can get those from the following:

- ✓ Mexican oregano
- ✓ flax seed
- ✓ dark chocolate
- ✓ dried rosemary
- ✓ black olives
- ✓ blueberries, raspberries, strawberries, elderberries, and blackberries

Natural Antibiotics For Acid Reflux

In several individuals, some foods can trigger the lower esophageal sphincter, letting the acid and food to go up into the esophagus.

This can give you some esophageal injury and other digestive problems. The following are some of the natural antibiotics that you can take to treat that acid reflux easily.

- ✓ Cabbage
- ✓ Banana
- ✓ Baking soda
- ✓ Cucumber

Whenever I consume those natural antibiotics my heartburn and indigestion are completely resolved which makes me feel much better.

Chapter 4 – Amazing Natural Antibiotics to Heal Wounds

Open wounds are usually painful and nasty not only are they are undesirable but needs a lot of waiting time to entirely heal. As a matter of fact, they usually leave a scar on your skin. This is a compilation of natural antibiotics to guarantee rapid recovery and get rid of any infection.

This is the primary reason why an individual has to keep in mind that the wound must keep from being infected that stops the recovery process. Putting up over-the-counter ointments on the lesion may or might not support the lesion to recover, but several ingredients that can be found at home might be a natural antibiotic that will work like a charm.

Yes, it is true, several ingredients that are usually utilized in our foods can become rejuvenators thus we loved their healing content. If you have not aware of these ingredients, we will tackle it down. These natural antibiotics will support you in cleaning your wound and give it an assurance that it will not get infected. Give it a guarantee that you will utilize them on a daily basis to get the best outcome.

Remember that these natural antibiotics are perfect to mix with treatments on nonserious wounds. Here are the natural antibiotics that you should consider immediately of taking if there is a presence of wounds.

✓ **Honey**

Putting it on an open laceration supports the draining of the bacteria from the wound and preventing the wound to get infected and inflamed. It is also recognized for its anti-fungal, anti-inflammatory, and anti-bacterial content. Put honey straightforwardly on the laceration every day before rinsing it.

✓ **Echinacea**

It has been utilized to cure infections for a long time already. Various herbal healers have utilized echinacea for lots of years to cure wounds. Experts are starting to have a grasp on the subject matter. S. pyogenes is known for toxic shock syndrome, sore throat, and other types of diseases.

Echinacea might combat inflammation as well linked with an infection that is due to bacteria. It can be purchased easily because it is widely available.

✓ **Turmeric**

This simple ingredient has antibacterial properties that have been utilized for a long time already to treat various issues in our health. The so-called curcumin in it supports in promoting wound recovery by building collagen. If the laceration is bleeding, put the turmeric on it to end bleeding. You can also consume turmeric milk before bedtime to quicken up the process of healing.

✓ **Limestone powder**

It is also recognized as the term chuna which is usually utilized in paan, has healing content. Just get turmeric and chuna and cook them and put the solution on the laceration as it will surely support wound recovery.

✓ **Aloe Vera**

It has anti-inflammatory, analgesic, and rejuvenating content that will quicken up the healing time. It also has phytochemicals that will lessen the pain and prevent inflammation. Slice an aloe vera leaf and get the gel. Put the gel on the laceration and allow it to dry. Sanitize the area with warm water and wipe it down with a dry cloth.

✓ **Coconut oil**

It supports to lessen the pain and prevents infection. This is because of its anti-inflammatory, moisturizing, and anti-bacterial content. Also, it prevents the accumulation of scar as well. Just put this oil on the wound and put some bandage on it. To quicken up healing you must put this oil 2 to 3 times a day.

✓ **Onion**

It has an anti-bacterial compound called allicin that secures the laceration from infection. To do that put honey and onion in a blender to make a batter. Put it straightforwardly on the wound to cut down healing time.

With these natural antibiotics, you will not have any problems at all in healing those wounds and as a matter of fact, you will not be exposed to lots of artificial chemicals that can make you prone to side-effects.

I have been using those natural antibiotics whenever I get wounds even though it is minor or serious. I only seek help from a medical professional if the wounds did not heal for almost two days that is why these natural antibiotics are worth the try and will surely save you a lot of money and time going to the doctor.

Conclusion

Now you know, that there are lots of natural antibiotics that are available in your house. You will now have the ability to lessen the side-effects of artificial antibiotics that is why you do not have any reasons at all not to get healed. So the next time you have a health issue that you want to get rid either it's a simple wound or experiencing serious viral infection then you might want to try this natural intervention as well.

Always get a feel of yourself if your condition is improving however if you feel that you are not getting well then there is nothing much better than seeking a doctor's advice. However, most of the time there is a large percentage that your illnesses will be resolved with these natural antibiotics except that there is an underlying problem besides your infection.

Either you will use it for your wounds, viral infection, stomach problems, and other medical conditions you must always take these natural antibiotics into mind. So try these natural antibiotics whenever you need to and expect that you will have a much more desirable healing experience compared to the artificial antibiotics.